The Easy and Professional Low-Carb Cookbook

Simple & Satisfying Recipes for a Healthy Diet

Jamie S. Garner

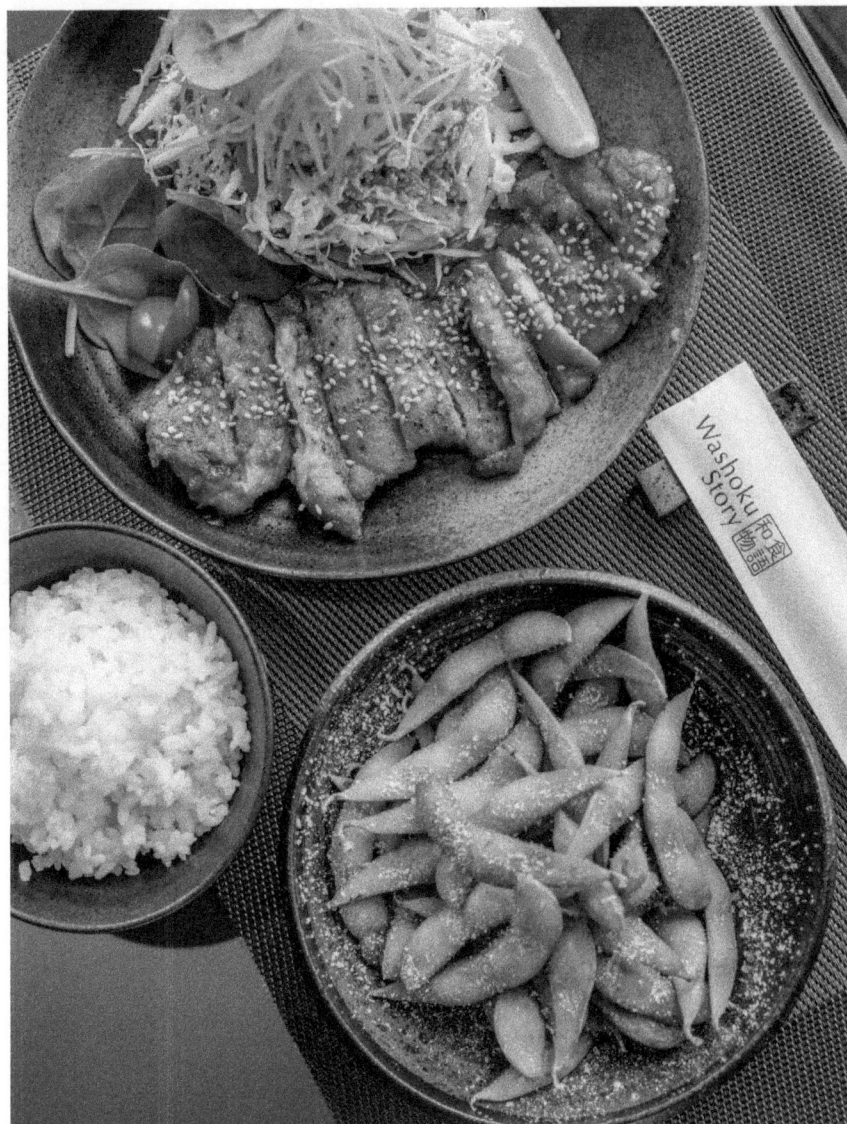

Table Of Contents

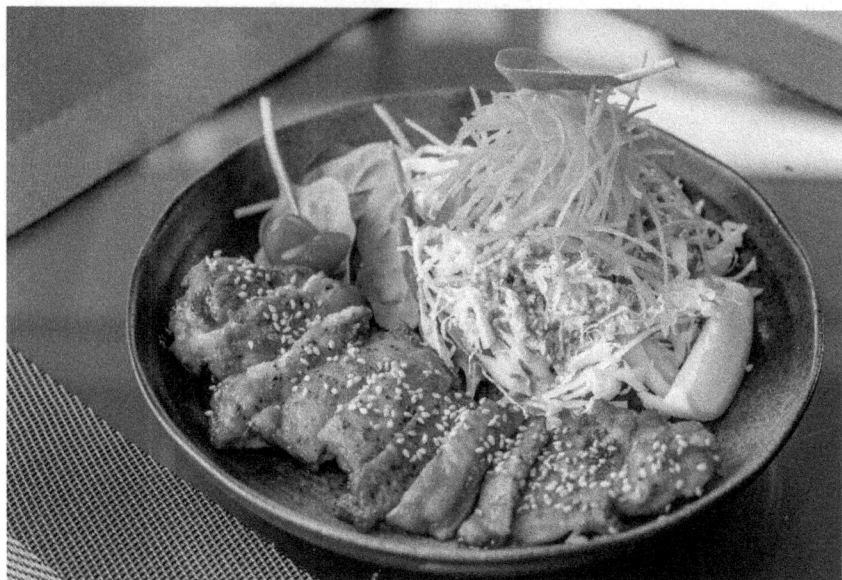

Margaret King's Tortilla Chips

You can buy low-carb tortilla chips, but there's a charm to fresh ones.

Low-carb tortillas

Nonstick cooking spray

Spray the tortillas with cooking spray, both sides, and cut them into triangle

shapes. Bake on a cookie sheet at 400°F (200°C) for 10 to 15 minutes, until

crisp and brown. They make great dippers for all chip and dip needs!

Tester's note: Barbo Gold, who tested these, liked them the way Margaret made

them, but thought they were even better baked at 250°F (130°C) for 1 hour and

10 minutes. She also suggests a sprinkle of salt, and even onion powder. Knock

you rself out.

Each whole tortilla has: 50 calories; 2 g fat; 5 g

protein; 11 g carbohydrate;

8 g dietary fiber; 3 g usable carbs.

Jill Taylor's Fried Cheese Taco Shells

Who could miss those stale corn ones, out of a box?

1 8-ounce (225 g) bag of shredded Mexican 4-Cheese blend

Don't use fat-free cheese!

Heat a small nonstick skillet over medium heat until hot. Add 1;'2 cup (30 g) of

shredded cheese and fry until brown. Flip over and brown the other side. Do not

overcook as it becomes dry and brittle. Light golden brown is good. When

cooked, remove from the skillet and place over a rolling pin covered with a

kitchen towel. Use another folded piece of kitchen towel to mold the cheese into

a taco shape, then put aside to cool. Always wipe the excess fat from the pan

before you add more cheese, as it cooks better if it is dry.

If you prefer nachos to tacos, cook the cheese the same way but place flat on a

piece of kitchen towel when cooked and cut into "chips" with a pizza cutter

before it is cold.

YIELD: Makes 8 tortilla shells or rounds to cut up

Each having: 114 calories; 9 g fat; 7 g protein; trace carbohydrate; no fiber, trace

usable carbs.

Mindy Sauve's Low-Carb Nachos Supreme

A fast, teen-friendly dinner!

1 pound (455 g) low-fat ground beef

1 15-ounce (420 g) can Eden Black Soy Beans, drained

1 7 3/4-ounce (220 g) can Mexican Hot-Style Tomato Sauce (if you can't

find this, use regular tomato sauce with 3 tablespoons (45 ml) enchilada

sauce added!)

1 12-ounce (340 g) bag Soy and Flaxseed Tortilla Chips (or make own

chips from Margaret King's Tortilla Chips (page 70)

2 cups (240 g) grated Mexican Cheese blend (or cheese of choice)

1 7 3/4-ounce (220 g) can sliced black olives

1 tomato, diced

Sour cream to taste

Brown and crumble ground beef, and drain fat. Add black soy beans and Mexican

tomato sauce. Cook just until all heated through.

Spread the contents of a bag of low-carb chips on a plate; top with 1j4 cup

(30 g) grated cheese. Spoon 1j2 cup (60 g) meat/bean mixture on top. Top meat

mixture with another 1j4 cup (30 g) cheese. Sprinkle with olives. Microwave the

whole thing on high for 45 seconds until cheese is melted.

Top with chopped tomato and sour cream to taste.

Dana's note: I might use Pat Best' Refried Black Soy Beans (page 63) instead of

the plain black soy beans.

YIELD: Serves 8 or more

Each has: 517 calories; 39 g fat (61.2% calories from fat); 30 g protein;

25 g carbohydrate; 16 g dietary fiber; 9 g usable

carbs.

Susan Higgs's Salmon Stuffed Celery

A great party snack or sack lunch.

1 15-ounce (420 g) can salmon, drained,

or 2 vacuum-packed packages salmon

8 ounces (225 g) softened cream cheese

Juice and zest of one lemon

1 teaspoon prepared horseradish

1 tablespoon (10 g) dried minced onion flakes

'/4 teaspoon salt

1 tablespoon (15 ml) Worcestershire sauce (you may want to add this

1 teaspoon at a time, depending on how well you like the

Worcestershire sauce)

1 bunch celery, cut in thirds

Mix all ingredients together except celery. Chill for 4 to 8 hours.

Stuff salmon-cheese mixture into celery thirds and

serve.

Yield: 20 servings

Each has: 71 calories; 5 g fat; 5 g protein; 1 g carbohydrate; trace dietary fiber;

1 g usable carbs.

Herbert D. Focken's Sweetened

Jalapeno Bites

Our tester, Julie, called this "really interesting, and surprisingly good!" (She also

said it really improved low-carb crackers, of which she is not generally fond.)

1 12-ounce (340 g) jar sliced jalapeno peppers

3/4 cup (18 g) Splenda

Cream cheese-plain or onion-chive flavored

Pork rinds or low-carb crackers

Dump out the jalapenos, including the liquid, into a bowl, and stir in the Splenda.

Pack them back into the jar, put on the lid, and stick it in the fridge for a day

or two.

When snack time rolls around, pull out the jar and grab your cream cheese and

pork rinds or low-carb crackers. Spread some cream

cheese on a pork rind or

cracker, top with a slice or two of jalapeno, and stuff it in your face! Repeat.

Your whole jar of sweetened peppers has the following: 94 calories; 2 g fat;

4 g protein; 18 g carbohydrate; 9 g dietary fiber; 9 g usable carbs. Working out

the per-piece counts of this was just too darned difficult, so we gave up-but

cream cheese is very low carb, and pork rinds are carb-free. If you're using low   carb crackers, read the label.

Linda Guiffre's Pizza Muffin Appetizers

Leftovers-if there are any-can be eaten cold the next day for lunch.

1-2 tablespoons (15-30 ml) olive oil

1 clove garlic, minced

'/2 cup (75 g) chopped green pepper

'/2 cup (75 g) chopped red pepper

'/2 small onion, chopped

1 cup (100 g) chopped mushrooms

'/4 cup (25 g) chopped olives

'/4_ V2 teaspoon red pepper flakes, or to taste

'/2 teaspoon Italian seasoning

Dash black pepper

2 eggs

2;'3 cup (100 g) grated Parmesan cheese

1 V2 cups (180 g) shredded mozzarella

8 ounces (225 g) cream cheese, softened

Approximately 30 slices of deli-sized pepperoni

'/2 cup (120 g) pizza sauce (optional)

In the olive oil saute the garlic, peppers, and onion until almost soft. Add the

mushrooms and saute a minute or two more. Turn off the heat and add the olives,

red pepper flakes, Italian seasoning, and pepper.

In a bowl, lightly beat your eggs, then add the Parmesan, mozzarella, and cream

cheese. Add your sauteed vegetables and mix all ingredients until blended.

Line each mini-muffin cup with a slice of pepperoni (forming a basket). Use a

teaspoon to drop the vegetable-cheese mixture into the pepperoni cup.

Bake for 25 minutes at 325 °F (170°C) or until very lightly browned.

If desired, serve with a bit of pizza sauce on top (may top each muffin with sauce

10 minutes prior to end of baking time, then return to oven to finish baking-or

simply top muffins with sauce when done), but they're good plain, too.

Yield: Makes about 30 mini-muffin-sized bites

Each with: 98 calories; 8 g fat; 4 g protein; 2 g carbohydrate; trace dietary fiber;

2g usable carbs.

Nancy Harrigan's Spinach Balls

Our tester, Patty Mishler, rated this a 10!

3 boxes, 10 ounces (280 g) each, frozen chopped spinach, thawed and

squeezed dry

2 cups (250 g) almond meal

1 V2 cups (185 g) chopped macadamia nuts

1 teaspoon salt

'/4 teaspoon garlic powder

2 tablespoons (20 g) dried minced onion

'/2 cup (80 g) grated Parmesan cheese

2 eggs or 4 egg whites

1 stick butter, melted

Mix together and form into 1" (2.5 cm) balls.

Bake ats 350°F (180 °C) for 20 min.

These may be baked dry and served with hollandaise sauce or a mustard sauce as an hors d' oeuvres. The balls should be bite-sized for this. Or you can bake these

in Nancy Harrigan's Coconut Ginger Sauce (page 445).

Nancy's note: "I like to bake these in the Coconut Ginger Sauce (page 445). Mix

the sauce and pour over balls before baking. This sauce will need to be doubled

for the whole batch of Spinach Balls. I bake them in this sauce (using butter) with

raw shrimp. Add a salad and you've got a fabulous dinner!

"I also like to make up the whole batch, put the balls on a cookie sheet, and

freeze them, then put them in a freezer bag and take them out as needed."

Yield: About 8 servings (6 balls each)

Each with: 464 calories; 38 g fat; 20 g protein; 17 g carbohydrate; 6 g dietary

fiber; 11 g usable carbs. Analysis does not include

any sauce or dip.

Audra Olsen's Asparagus/Salami Roll-Ups

1 pound (455 g) fresh or frozen asparagus

1 pound (455 g) hard salami, the smaller round ones

4 ounces (115 g) cream cheese

If you're using fresh asparagus, snap the end off each spear where it breaks natu rally, then plunge into boiling water for just 20 to 30 seconds; drain. If using

frozen asparagus, just thaw it.

Preheat oven to 375 °F (190°C) degrees.

Layout a slice of salami, spread with cream cheese, and place an asparagus spear

on one end, rolling it up. Seal with a dab of cream cheese and lay on a cookie

sheet. Once all processed, bake for 20 minutes. Serve.

Yield: Serves 4

Each serving will have: 397 calories; 33 g fat; 19 g protein; 6 g carbohydrate; 1 g

dietary fiber; 5 g usable carbs.

Eggs, Cheese,

and the Like

I've said it before, I'll say it again: eggs are not just for breakfast! They're one of

the most versatile foods we have in our low-carb diet, and for the protein they

offer-with almost no waste-they're a heckuva bargain. Better yet, many egg

recipes are fast! So have a dozen eggs-or more-in the fridge at all times.

We're also including recipes that get their protein from cheese in this chap ter, just because it seemed like a good idea. One of the best things about cheese is

that it keeps well. Further, it doesn't need defrosting. And all you have to do is heat

it up to make it seem like a meal, instead of a snack.

Of course, if you're a low-carb vegetarian, eggs and cheese will be among the staples of your diet. But everyone can enjoy meals centered around eggs and

cheese!

There are also some recipes in this chapter that involve substantial quantities

of things like sausage, ham, or bacon, along with the eggs and cheese. It was sort

of a judgment call, you know?

Here, repeated from two previous books, is the single skill I'm determined to

teach every low carber:

Dana's Easy Omelet Method

If I had to choose just one skill to teach to every new low carber, it would be how

to make an omelet. They're fast, they're easy, and they make a wide variety of sim   ple ingredients seem like a meal!

First, have your filling ready. If you're using vegetables, you'll want to saute them first. If you're using cheese, have it grated or sliced and ready to go. If you're

making an omelet to use up leftovers-a great idea, by the way-warm them

through in the microwave and have them standing by.

77 Spray your omelet pan well with cooking spray if it doesn't have a good

nonstick surface, and put it over medium-high heat. While the skillet's heat   ing, grab your eggs-2 is the perfect number for this size pan, but 1 or 3 will

work-and a bowl, crack the eggs, and beat them with a fork. Don't add any

water or milk or anything, just mix them up.

The pan is hot enough when a drop of water thrown in sizzles right away.

Add a tablespoon of oil or butter, slosh it around to cover the bottom, then

pour in the eggs, all at once. They should sizzle, too, and immediately start to set. When the bottom layer of egg is set around the edges-this should hap   pen quite quickly-lift the edge using a spatula and tip the pan to let the raw

egg flow underneath. Do this all around the edges, until there's not enough

raw egg to run.

Now, turn your burner to the lowest heat if you have a gas stove. If you

have an electric stove, you'll have to have a "warm" burner standing by;

electric elements don't cool off fast enough for this job. Put your filling on

one-half of the omelet, cover it, and let it sit over very low heat for a minute or

two, no more. Peek and see if the raw, shiny egg is gone from the top surface

(although you can serve it that way if you like-that's how the French prefer

their omelets), and the cheese, if you've used it, is melted. If not, re-cover the pan and let it go another minute or two.

When your omelet is done, slip a spatula under the half without the filling

and fold it over; then lift the whole thing onto a plate. Or you can get fancy and

tip the pan, letting the filling side of the omelet slide onto the plate, folding

the top over as you go, but this takes some practice.

This makes a single-serving omelet. I think it's a lot easier to make sever   al individual omelets than to make one big one, and omelets are so fast to

make that it's not that big a deal. Anyway, that way you can customize your

omelets to each individual's taste. If you're making more than 2 or 3 omelets,

just keep them warm in your oven, set to its very lowest heat.

Now here are some ideas for what to put in your omelets!

Club Omelet

One of the few high-carb meals I miss is the turkey club sandwich-so here's

the omelet equivalent!

2 slices bacon, cooked and drained

2 ounces (55 g) turkey breast slices

'/2 small tomato, sliced

1 scallion, sliced

2 eggs

1 tablespoon (15 g) mayonnaise

Have your bacon cooked and drained-I like to microwave mine and crumble it

up. Cut the turkey into small squares, and have the tomato and scallion sliced

and at hand.

Beat the eggs, and make your omelet according to Dana's Easy Omelet Method

(page 77), adding just the bacon and turkey while

it's still cooking. Then add the

tomato and scallion, spread the mayo on the other side, fold, and serve.

Yield: 1 serving

Each with: 383 calories; 28 g fat; 29 g protein; 5 g carbohydrate; 1 g dietary

fiber; 4 g usable carbs.

Mexican Avocado and Ham Omelet

This is actually a fairly traditional combination in Mexico.

1 pinch paprika

'/4 teaspoon salt

2 tablespoons (30 g) sour cream

2 eggs

'/4 cup (30 g) ham, minced

2 tablespoons (25 g) diced tomato

'/2 avocado, sliced

Have everything cut up before you start cooking. Stir the paprika and salt into

the sour cream.

Now, make your omelet according to Dana's Easy Omelet Method (page 77).

When bottom is set, add ham and tomato, cover the skillet, and set the burner to

low. Let it cook for a minute or two until top is set.

Arrange avocado slices on the

ham and tomato, fold omelet, and top with seasoned sour cream to serve.

Yield: 1 serving

Each with: 509 calories; 42 g fat; 23 g protein; 12 g carbohydrate; 3 g dietary

fiber; 9 g usable carbs.

Roman Mushroom Omelet

Believe it or not, this is classical Italian food, with no pasta in sight.

2 cups (200 g) sliced mushrooms

'/4 small onion, sliced thin

1 stalk celery, diced fine

2 tablespoons (30 ml) olive oil

1 clove garlic

'/2 teaspoon chicken bouillon concentrate

'/2 teaspoon Splenda

Salt and pepper

4 eggs

'/2 cup (80 g) shredded Romano cheese

80 Eggs, Cheese, and the Like In your big skillet, start sauteing the mushrooms, onion, and celery in the olive

oil. When the mushrooms have changed color and the onion is translucent, add the garlic, chicken bouillon granules, and Splenda, stirring till the bouillon dis   solves. Let cook for another minute or so. Salt and pepper the mushroom mixture

to taste, and remove from skillet.

Now, in your omelet pan, make 2 omelets, one after the other, according to

Dana's Easy Omelet Method (page 77), using the mushrooms as filling, with 1j4

cup (40 g) of shredded Romano cheese on top. Cover and cook till cheese melts,

fold, and serve. (You can keep the first omelet warm long enough to make the

second omelet by simply covering the plate with a spare pot lid. For that matter,

you can halve this recipe to make one omelet!)

Yield: 2 omelets

Each with: 388 calories; 30 g fat; 22 g protein; 8 g carbohydrate; , g dietary

fiber; 7 g usable carbs.

Sloppy Tom Omelet

I like this omelet as a quick lunch. Indeed, I've been known to make Sloppy

Toms just to have them on hand for this purpose. If you have a favorite low-carb

Sloppy Joe recipe, feel free to use it instead.

2 eggs

1j4 cup (50 g) Sloppy Toms (page 259)

, ounce (30 g) cheddar cheese or Monterey Jack, sliced or shredded

If your Sloppy Toms are left over, straight out of the fridge, warm them a bit in

the microwave before you start cooking the eggs. Then make your omelet

according to Dana's Easy Omelet Method (page 77), adding the cheese first,

then the Sloppy Toms on top of the cheese. Cover, turn burner to low, and finish

cooking, then fold and serve.

Yield: , serving

Each with: 346 calories; 23 g fat; 27 g protein; 7 g carbohydrate; , g dietary

fiber; 6 g usable carbs.

81 ~ Ropa Vieja Omelet

Here's another way to use your Ropa Vieja (page 319)

'/3 cup (70 g) Ropa Vieja

1 ounce (30 g) Monterey Jack cheese

'/4 California avocado, sliced

2 eggs

Warm your Ropa Vieja in the microwave, slice or shred your cheese, and slice

your avocado; have everything standing by!

Now heat your omelet pan, and add a little oil.

When it's time to add the filling, put the cheese in first, then the Ropa Vieja,

then the avocado. Cover, turn burner to low, and

finish cooking, then fold and

serve.

Yield: 1 serving

Each with: 445 calories; 34 g fat; 29 g protein; 5 g carbohydrate; 2 g dietary

fiber; 3 g usable carbs.

Machaca Eggs

True Machaca is made with beef that you've salted and dried, then rehydrated in

boiling water, and pounded into shreds. It's very tasty, but I don't know a lot of

people who want to do that much work. The beef shreds from the Ropa Vieja

work beautifully in this scramble!

2 tablespoons (30 ml) olive oil

1 cup (200 g) Ropa Vieja (page 319)

'/2 green bell pepper, diced

'/2 onion, chopped

1 clove garlic, crushed

1 cup (225 g) canned tomatoes with green chilies, drained

5 eggs

'/4 cup (20 g) chopped fresh cilantro

Heat the olive oil in a large, heavy skillet, and add

the Ropa Vieja, diced pepper

and onion, and the garlic. Saute them together, stirring often, until the onion and

pepper are becoming a little soft. In the meanwhile, measure your tomatoes and

scramble up your eggs.

Okay, your onion is translucent, and your pepper's starting to soften. Add the

tomato, stir it up, then pour in the beaten eggs. Scramble until the eggs are set.

Divide evenly between two plates, top each serving with half the cilantro, and

serve.

Feel free to add some chopped jalapenos or more green chilies to this, if

you'd like it spicy. Or you could use a pasilla or Anaheim chili in place of the

green pepper.

Yield: 2 to3 servings

Assuming 2 servings, each will have: 520 calories; 39 g fat; 30 g protein;

12 g carbohydrate; 2 g dietary fiber; 10 g usable carbs.

Italian Sausage and Mushroom Scramble

2 ounces (55 g) Italian sausage link

1 tablespoon (15 ml) olive oil

3/4 cup (75 g) chopped mushrooms

2 tablespoons (16 g) grated carrot

1 scallion

3 eggs

2 tablespoons (20 g) grated Parmesan cheese

Slice the sausage down the middle the long way, then lay flat side down and slice

into half-rounds, about '/4" (6.25 mm) thick. Heat the olive oil in a large skillet,

over medium-low heat, and start browning the sausage.

In the meanwhile, cut up your mushrooms, grate your carrot, and slice your scal   lion. When the sausage is browned on the first side, turn it over, and add the veg   gies. Cook, stirring now and then, until the mushrooms soften a bit.

Beat the eggs with the Parmesan, and pour over the sausage and vegetables.

Scramble till set, and serve.

Yield: 1 to 2 servings

Assuming 1 serving, it will have: 582 calories; 48 g fat; 30 g protein;

7 g carbohydrate; 1 g dietary fiber; 6 g usable carbs.

Spring Ham and Mushroom Scramble

Ham and eggs scrambled together are nothing new- it's the seasoning that

makes this taste fresh as springtime!

'/2 cup (50 g) sliced mushrooms

'/2 cup (55 g) ham cubes

1 teaspoon butter

4 eggs

3/4 teaspoon dried dill weed

'/2 teaspoon lemon juice

4 scallions, sliced V4" (6.25 mm) thick

84 Eggs, Cheese, and the Like In a small-to-medium-sized nonstick skillet, start sauteing the mushrooms and

ham cubes in the butter. While that's happening, scramble your eggs with the dill

and lemon.

When the mushrooms are limp and have changed

color, add the eggs and sliced

scallions to the skillet. Scramble till eggs are set, and serve.

Yield: 2 servings

Each with: 225 calories; 14 g fat; 18 g protein; 5 g carbohydrate; 1 g dietary

fiber; 4 g usable carbs.

Springtime Scramble

4 stalks asparagus

8 fresh snow pea pods

1 scallion

3 eggs

1 teaspoon olive oil

Snap the bottoms off your asparagus where they break naturally, then cut the

stalks into V2" (1 .25 cm) pieces, on the diagonal. Pinch the ends off the snow

peas, and pull off the strings, then cut them into '/2" (1 .25 cm) pieces, too. Put

the two in a microwaveable bowl, add just a couple of teaspoons of water, cover,

and microwave on high for just 3 minutes. Uncover as soon as the microwave

beeps! While this is happening, slice your scallion, including the crisp part of the

green, and beat up your eggs.

Okay, pull your asparagus and snow peas out of the microwave. Spray a medium

skillet with nonstick cooking spray, and place over medium heat. Add the olive

oil, and let it start heating. Drain the asparagus and snow peas, and throw 'em in

the skillet, along with the scallion. Now pour in the eggs, and scramble till set.

That's it!

Yield: 1 serving

Each with: 267 calories; 18 g fat; 19 g protein; 8 g carbohydrate; 2 g dietary

fiber; 6 g usable carbs.

Marilee Wellersdick's Bean Sprout Scramble

Like bean sprouts? They're very low carb and quite good for you.

2 tablespoons (30 g) butter

1 tablespoon (10 g) minced onion

'/2 cup (25 g) bean sprouts

3 eggs

Salt and pepper

1 tablespoon (15 g) sour cream (optional)

Melt the butter in a nonstick skillet. Add the onion and sprouts and stir until the

sprouts are tender crisp (onions should be translucent by then). Scramble the

eggs, add salt and pepper, and add them to the skillet, stirring the mixture until

the eggs are set. To serve, top with a dollop of sour cream, if desired.

Yield: This recipe is for 1 serving

Assuming 1 serving, each will have: 550 calories; 40 g fat; 18 g protein;

6 g carbohydrate; 2 g dietary fiber; 4 g usable carbs.

Quiche Lorraine

Quiche has somehow acquired a reputation for being foofy, girly food-but it's

entirely made of stuff men love! So tell your husband this is "Bacon, Egg, and

Cheese Pie," and watch him yum it down.

1 Pie Crust, unbaked (page 132)

8 ounces (225 g) Gruyere cheese

12 slices bacon

5 eggs

'/2 cup (120 ml) Carb Countdown Dairy Beverage

'/2 cup (120 ml) heavy cream or you can use 1 cup (240 ml)

half-and-half in place of the Carb Countdown and the cream

1 pinch ground nutmeg

1 tablespoon (15 ml) dry vermouth

'/2 teaspoon salt or Vege-Sal

'/4 teaspoon pepper

Have your crust ready in the pan and standing by.

Preheat oven to 350°F (180°C).

Shred your cheese, and cook and drain your bacon-I microwave my bacon, and I

find that 1 minute per slice on high is about right, but your microwave may be a

little different.

First put the cheese in the pie shell, covering the bottom evenly. Crumble the

bacon evenly over the cheese.

Now whisk together the eggs, Carb Countdown Dairy Beverage, cream, nutmeg,

vermouth, salt, and pepper. Pour this over the cheese and bacon. Bake for 45

minutes, then cool. It's actually traditional to serve Quiche Lorraine at room

temperature, but you certainly may warm it if you like.

Yield: 8 servings

Each with: 470 calories; 37 g fat; 32 g protein; 4 g carbohydrate;

1 g dietary fiber; 3 g usable carbs.

Spinach Mushroom Quiche

1 Almond-Parmesan Crust, prebaked (page 132)

8 ounces (225 g) sliced mushrooms

'/2 cup (80 g) chopped onion

2 tablespoons (30 g) butter

10 ounces (280 g) frozen chopped spinach, thawed

3 eggs

3/4 cup (175 ml) heavy cream

3/4 cup (175 ml) Carb Countdown Dairy Beverage

2 tablespoons (30 ml) dry vermouth

'/2 teaspoon salt

'/4 teaspoon pepper

1 V2 cups (180 g) shredded Monterey Jack cheese

Have your crust ready first.

In a large, heavy skillet, over medium-high heat, saute the mushrooms and onion in

the butter until the onion is translucent and the

mushrooms are limp. Transfer into

a large mixing bowl, preferably one with a pouring lip.

Dump your thawed spinach into a strainer, and using clean hands, squeeze all the

moisture out of it you can. Add it to the mushrooms and onions.

Now add the eggs, cream, and Carb Countdown Dairy Beverage. Whisk the whole

thing up until well combined. Whisk in the vermouth, salt, and pepper.

Cover the bottom of the Almond-Parmesan Crust with the Monterey Jack, and put

it in the oven at 325 °F (170 °C) for just a couple of minutes, or until the cheese

just starts to melt. Take it out of the oven, and pour in the egg-vegetable mix ture-your quiche will be very full! Very carefully place it back in the oven. It's a

good idea to place a flat pan under it, on the floor

of the oven, to catch any drips.

Bake for 50 to 60 minutes, or until just set in the center. Let cool. Quiche is

traditionally served at room temperature, but if you like it warm, it's better to make

this ahead, let it cool, and even chill it, then cut slices and warm them for

a minute or two on 70 percent power in your microwave, rather than serving it

right out of the oven.

Yield: 8 servings

Each with: 480 calories; 43 g fat; 17 g protein; 10 g carbohydrate; 4 g dietary

fiber; 6 g usable carbs.

73

Deb Gajewski's Zucchini Quiche

Our tester, Linda, thought this was a very tasty recipe-even her husband, no

big fan of vegetables, liked this.

2 cups (240 g) zucchini, cut in thin half-rounds

2 tablespoons (30 g) butter

12 cherry tomatoes

2 tablespoons (15 g) low-carb bake mix

2 extra large eggs

3/4 cup (180 g) yogurt

1 teaspoon oregano

8 ounces (225 g) cream cheese, Kraft '/3 less fat

'/3 cup (50 g) Parmesan cheese

Preheat oven to 375 °F (190°C). Spray a 9" (22.5 cm) pie plate with nonstick

cooking spray.

In your big, heavy skillet, saute the zucchini in the butter until it's limp. Add the tomatoes. Cook for 3 more minutes. Cool for 5 to 10 minutes. Stir in the low   carb bake mix and spoon the whole thing into buttered 9" (22.5 cm) pie plate.

In a separate bowl, lightly beat your eggs. Add the yogurt and oregano, then

whisk in the cream cheese in small bits. Mix together lightly. Spoon on top of the

vegetables, and sprinkle the Parmesan on top.

Bake for 30 minutes at 375 °F (190°C) or until firm in center. Serve.

Yield: Makes 4 servings

Each with: 333 calories; 25 g fat; 17 g protein; 9 g carbohydrate; 2 g dietary

fiber; 7 g usable carbs.

Sausage Mushroom Quiche

Serve this with a salad on the side, and warm up any leftovers for breakfast.

1 pound (445 g) bulk sausage, hot or mild as you prefer

1 cup (160 g) chopped white onions

1 cup (100 g) sliced fresh mushrooms

4 eggs plus 1 egg yolk, lightly beaten

'/2 teaspoon Dijon mustard

'/2 teaspoon dry mustard

'/8 teaspoon cayenne pepper

'/8 teaspoon nutmeg

1 cup (120 g) shredded Monterey Jack cheese

1 cup (150 g) grated Parmesan

2 cups (480 ml) heavy cream

1 teaspoon chopped parsley

Preheat your oven to 300°F (150 °C).

First, cook sausage, onions, and mushrooms together, crumbling the sausage,

until sausage is brown and vegetables cooked through. Drain, drain, drain.

(Jan usually pours off excess grease, then drains it further by placing mixture on

paper towels.) Press this mixture into the bottom of 10" (25 cm) pie plate

you've sprayed with nonstick spray. (Alternatively, our tester suggests a 9" x 13"

(22.5 x 32.5 cm) rectangular baking dish.)

Next, whisk together the 4 eggs and 1 yolk with the Dijon mustard, dry mustard,

cayenne pepper, nutmeg, Jack cheese, and 2/3 cup (100 g) of the Parmesan

cheese. Mix well.

Pour your cream into a heavy-bottomed saucepan, and put it over low heat.

Heat just to the boiling point (do not boil!). Then pour this scalded cream into

the egg mixture. Mix and pour custard over sausage crust in pie plate. Bake at

300°F (150°C) for around 35 minutes or until set. Sprinkle with remaining

Parmesan cheese and parsley. Let cool for 15 minutes before cutting.

Note: Jan says, "I've also used leftover chicken and broccoli in place of the

sausage and mushrooms. It's all good!"

Yield: 8 servings

Each will have: 591 calories; 55 g fat; 19 g protein; 5 g carbohydrate; trace

dietary fiber; 5 g usable carbs.

Tracie Jansen's Cheesy Spinach Pie

This would make a great brunch dish, or light supper, and could be a real ace in

the hole if you have vegetarians coming to dinner.

3 large eggs

1/2 cup (120 ml) heavy cream

1/4 teaspoon garlic powder

1/4 teaspoon Tabasco sauce

2 tablespoons (15 g) low-carb baking mix

Salt and pepper

1 V2 cups (180 g) shredded Cheddar cheese

1/4 cup (50 g) shredded Parmesan cheese

1 10-ounce (280 g) box frozen chopped spinach, thawed and well drained

Preheat oven to 350°F (180°C). Grease a 9" (22.5 cm) pie plate.

Whisk together the eggs, cream, garlic powder, Tabasco, baking mix, and salt and pepper.

Stir in cheeses and spinach until well combined. Pour mixture into prepared

pie plate.

Bake for approximately 35 minutes, or until set and starting to brown on top.

Let cool slightly, then cut into 8 wedges.

Tracie's note: "This recipe can be adapted many ways. For a Greek Spinach Pie,

add oregano and substitute feta cheese. I will use whatever cheese I have in the

fridge ... Swiss, blue, mozzarella ... or a combination of any of those."

Yield: About 8 servings

Each with: 188 calories; 15 g fat; 11 g protein; 3 g carbohydrate; 1 g dietary

fiber; 2 g usable carbs.

UnPotato Tortilla

Don't think Mexican flatbread, think eggs. In Spain, a "tortilla" is much like an

Italian frittata-a substantial egg dish, cooked in a skillet and served in wedges.

This one is my version of a traditional dish served in tapas bars all over Spain.

As bar food goes, it's a heckuva step up from beer nuts and stale popcorn!

'/4 head cauliflower

1 medium turnip

1 medium onion, sliced thin

3 tablespoons (45 ml) olive oil

6 eggs

Salt and pepper

Thinly slice your cauliflower-include the stem-and peel and thinly slice

your turnip. Put them in a microwaveable casserole with a lid, add a couple of tablespoons of water, and microwave on high for 6 to 7 minutes.

In the meanwhile, start the onion sauteing in 2 tablespoons (30 ml) of the olive

oil in an 8" (20 cm) to 9" (22.5 cm) skillet-a nonstick skillet is ideal, but not

essential. If your skillet isn't nonstick, give it a good squirt of nonstick cooking

spray first. Use medium heat.

When your microwave goes beep, pull out the veggies, drain them, and throw

them in the skillet with the onion. Continue sauteing everything, adding a bit

more oil if things start to stick, until the veggies are getting golden around the

edges-about 10 to 15 minutes. Turn the burner to low, and spread the vegeta   bles in an even layer on the bottom of the skillet.

Scramble up the eggs with a little salt and pepper, and pour over the vegetables.

Cook on low for 5 to 7 minutes, lifting the edges frequently to let uncooked egg

run underneath. When it's all set except for the top, slide the skillet under a low

broiler for 4 to 5 minutes, or until the top of your tortilla is golden. (If your skil   let doesn't have a flameproof handle, wrap it in foil first.) Cut in wedges to serve.

A little chopped parsley is nice on this, but not essential.

Yield: 6 servings

Each with: 139 calories; 11 g fat; 6 g protein; 4 g carbohydrate; 1 g dietary fiber;

3 g usable carbs.

Eliot Sohmer's Bacon Cheese Frittata

Y'know, it strikes me that this one is the epitome of the stereotype of low-carb

food-eggs, bacon, cheese. And a beautiful thing it is, too.

6 eggs

1 cup (240 ml) whole milk or Carb Countdown Dairy Beverage

2 tablespoons (30 g) butter, melted

'/2 teaspoon salt

'/4 teaspoon pepper

'/4 cup (25 g) chopped green onion

5 bacon strips, cooked and crumbled

1 cup (120 g) cheddar cheese, shredded

Preheat oven to 350°F (180°C). Spray an 7"-11" (27.5x17.5 cm) baking dish with

nonstick cooking spray.

In a mixing bowl, whisk together the eggs, milk or

Carb Countdown Dairy

Beverage, butter, salt, and pepper. Stir in the green onion, crumbled bacon, and

cheese. Pour into prepared dish, and bake, uncovered, for 25 to 30 minutes, or

until a knife inserted in center comes out clean.

Yield: Serves 6

Each with: 232 calories; 18 g fat; 13 g protein; 3 g carbohydrate; trace dietary

fiber; 3 g usable carbs.

Artichoke and Friends Frittata

3 tablespoons (45 ml) olive oil

'/4 pound (115 g) zucchini (about 1 really little zucchini), diced small

3 tablespoons (30 g) chopped onion

1 clove garlic, crushed

'/2 small green pepper, diced

'/2 small red pepper, diced

1 cup (300 g) canned artichoke hearts, drained and chopped

1 cup (110 g) '/4" (6.25 mm) ham cubes

'/4 cup (15 g) chopped fresh parsley

10 eggs

1 tablespoon (5 g) oregano

'/3 cup (50 g) grated Parmesan cheese

For this you need an oven-safe skillet-a big cast-iron skillet works great.

Spray the skillet with nonstick cooking spray, and

put it over medium-high heat.

Add the olive oil, and start sauteing the zucchini, onion, garlic, and peppers.

When the vegetables are starting to soften, stir in the artichoke hearts, ham

cubes, and fresh parsley. Let the whole thing continue cooking while you ...

Scramble up the eggs with the oregano and Parmesan.

Arrange the stuff in the skillet in an even layer, and pour in the eggs. Cover the

pan, turn the burner to low, and let the whole thing cook for 15 to 20 minutes,

or until all but the top is set.

Run the skillet under the broiler for 3 or 4 minutes until it starts to brown a little,

then cut frittata in wedges to serve.

Yield: 4 to 5 servings

Assuming 5 servings, each will have: 308 calories;

21 g fat; 20 g protein;

8 g carbohydrate; 1 g dietary fiber; 7 g usable carbs.

Savory Cheese and Ham Torte

This is great for any meal, both hot and cold. It even looks great! Our tester, Kim

Pulley, says this was "one of the best of the bunch."

1 10-ounce (280 g) package frozen chopped spinach

3 8-ounce (225 g) packages cream cheese, softened

'/2 cup (120 ml) heavy cream

1 tablespoon (15 g) Dijon mustard

'/2 tablespoon (10 g) salt

1 teaspoon (10 g) dried oregano

4 eggs

1 '/2 cups (180 g) shredded Swiss or Gruyere cheese

'/2_3/4 cup (55-80 g) diced ham

2 tablespoons (10 g) chopped fresh parsley

Preheat oven to 325 of (170°C). Grease a 9" (22.5 cm) springform pan.

Place your box of frozen spinach in the microwave

on a paper towel and cook on

high for 4 to 5 minutes. Carefully remove and drain, squeezing out most of the

moisture-it's good to dump it in a sieve and press it hard with the back of a

spoon. Set aside to cool.

In a large bowl, beat cream cheese and next 5 ingredients until smooth. Fold in

cheese, ham, parsley, and cooked spinach. Pour mixture into prepared pan. Bake

about 1 '/4 hours or until knife inserted in center of torte comes out clean. Cool

torte slightly in pan on wire rack. Cover and refrigerate until cold, about 3 hours.

To serve, run a thin knife blade around the edge, then carefully remove side of

pan. Cut torte into wedges.

Diane's note: I cut it into 12 wedges and heat in the microwave as needed when I want it warm, but it is equally delicious cold.

Yield: 12 wedges

Each will have: 327 calories; 30 g fat; 12 g protein; 3 g carbohydrate; trace

dietary fiber; 3 g usable carbs.

Eliot Sohmer's Spinach soume

This simple but great dish would be a fine side dish, but also would serve well

as a vegetarian entree. Our tester, Kay Winefordner, emphasizes the need to

drain the spinach very well!

2 cups (450 g) cottage cheese

3 eggs, beaten

3 10-ounce (280 g) packages frozen chopped spinach, thawed

2 cups (240 g) grated cheddar cheese

Salt to taste

Spray a 9" x 11" (22.5 x 2Z5 cm) baking pan with nonstick cooking spray.

Preheat your oven to 350°F (180°C).

Mix cottage cheese and eggs with spoon in mixing bowl. Drain your spinach very

well-it's best to dump it into a colander and press it hard with your hands or the back of a spoon, or even actually pick it up in handfuls and squeeze it hard!

Stir the spinach, 1 1;2 cups (180 g) of the cheddar, and salt if you like, into the

egg mixture. Pour into your prepared pan. Sprinkle the reserved cheddar cheese

on top. Bake 30 to 45 minutes at 350°F (180°C) until set.

Yield: Serves 6

Each getting: 276 calories; 16 g fat; 26 g protein; 9 g carbohydrate;

4 g dietary fiber; 5 g usable carbs.

96 Eggs, Cheese, and the Like ~ Betsy Calvin's Breakfast Casserole

This easy, crowd-pleasing brunch dish would also make a filling supper.

Our tester, Ray, who liked this a lot, suggested halving this recipe for

smaller groups.

1 pound (455 g) bulk Italian sausage (Betsy uses Bob Evan's brand)

5 cups (600 g) shredded sharp cheddar

12 eggs

1 cup (240 ml) heavy cream

Preheat oven to 325 °F (170°C). Spray an 9" X12" (22.5 x 30 cm) pan with

nonstick cooking spray.

First, cook and crumble your sausage, and drain it.

Spread 2 '/2 cups (300 g) of cheese in the prepared pan. Whisk your eggs in a

bowl, then pour on top of the cheese. Add the sausage, then the cream, and top

with the remaining cheese. Bake at 325 °F (170°C) for 45 minutes. Delicious!!!!

Yield: 8 servings

Each with: 683 calories; 59 g fat; 35 g protein; 3 g carbohydrate; 0 g dietary

fiber; 3 g usable carbs.

Stephanie H.'s French Toasty Eggs

This quick and easy microwave recipe makes eggs taste like a Danish. Our

tester, Ray, called this "fast and great"-a real treat you can make on a busy

morning!

2 ounces (55 g) cream cheese

2 eggs, lightly beaten

2 tablespoons (30 ml) sugar-free pancake syrup, divided

(do not use aspartame-sweetened syrup)

Ground cinnamon, to taste (careful, cinnamon is one of those

carb-y spices)

Soften the cream cheese in a microwave safe bowl, about 20 to 30 seconds on

high. Then add the eggs and 1 tablespoon (15 ml) of the syrup, stirring to mix.

This shouldn't mix completely; you'll have little bits

of cream cheese remaining.

Microwave for about a minute, then stir to break up any lumps. Microwave until

you have a large puffy pancakelike result; in my microwave this takes another

minute. Drizzle with remaining syrup and top with a few sprinkles of cinnamon.

Yield: Single serving

Each with: 331 calories; 29 g fat; 15 g protein; 3 g carbohydrate; trace dietary

fiber; 3 g usable carbs.

Cheese "Danish"

A contributor identified only as "Hihopesor" writes, "This is my version of a

Weight Watchers Danish with an English muffin, which of course has way too

many carbs. I used to fix this for my kids as breakfast before school but never

really appreciated just how good it probably was for them" Our tester, Ray, says

this is, "very quick, very easy, very good." What more could you want? Oh, yes   it's a good source of calcium, too!

1 slice low-carb bread, toasted and buttered

Up to 1;4 cup (60 g) cottage cheese, or as much as your toast will hold

Cinnamon to taste

Splenda to taste

Toast the bread, butter is optional; spread on the cottage cheese and sprinkle with cinnamon and Splenda. Put under the broiler until the cheese

starts to bubble.

Yield: 1 "Danish"

Carb count will depend on what brand of low-carb bread you use. To that,

add: 53 calories; 1 g fat; 8 g protein; 3 g carbohydrate; trace dietary fiber;

3 g usable carbs.

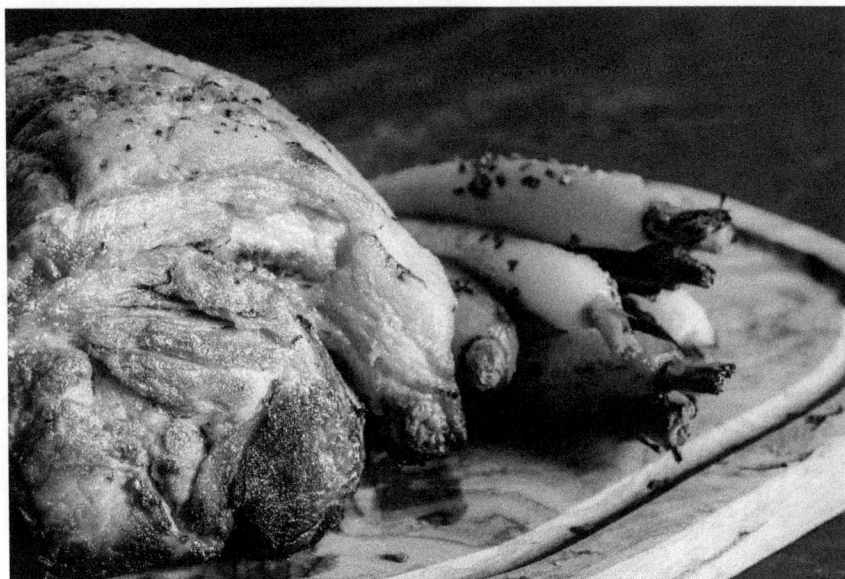

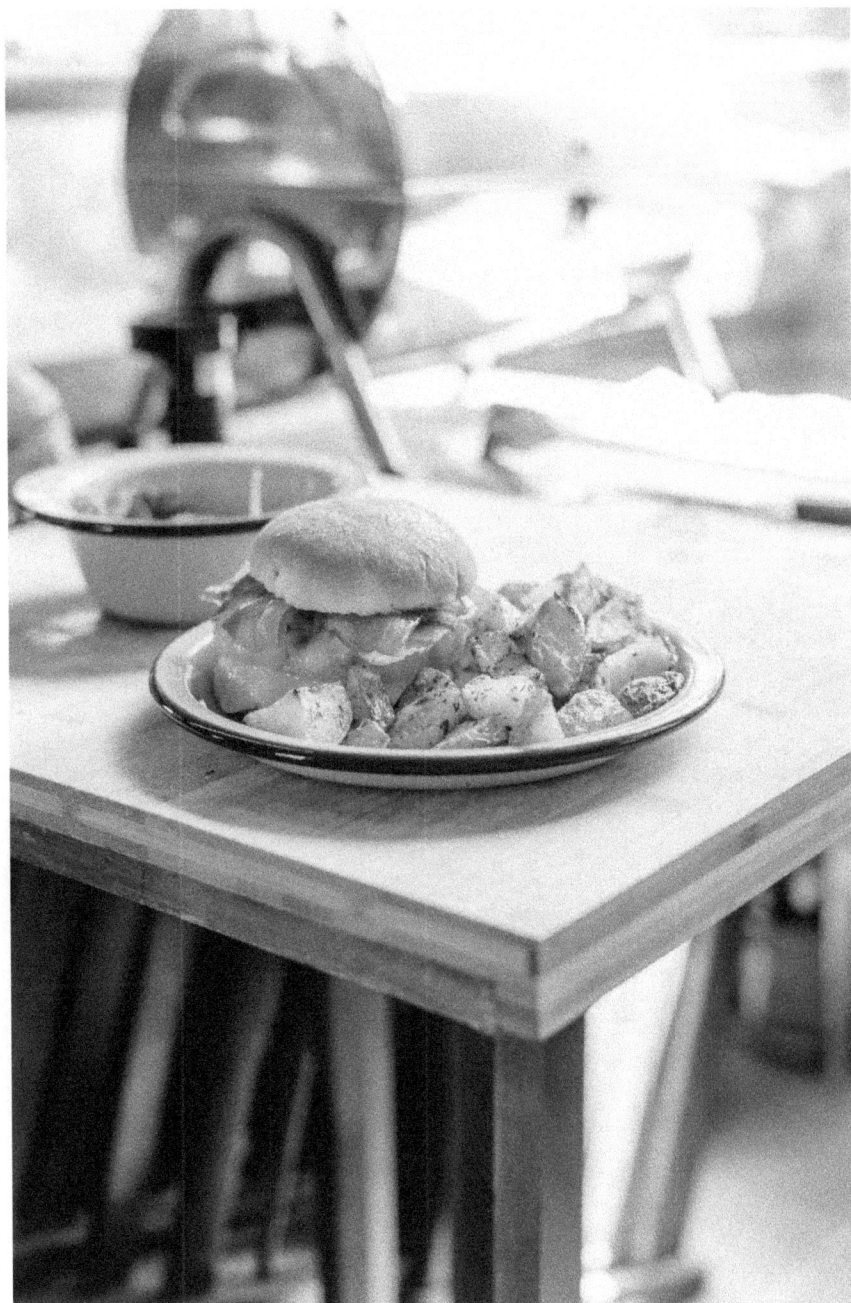

9 781802 832518